# Sleep;

**Get the Peaceful and Energising Sleep You Deserve, Sleeping Cures, Restless Sleep Syndrome, Insomnia, Sleeping Disorders**

**By**

**M Laurence**

*For Dianne to help with getting an amazing night's sleep*

# Chapters

# 1. Introduction

We all know how it feels when your alarm goes off first thing in the morning and you don't feel like you had any sleep. That's usually an odd occurrence for most people. Yes we feel terrible but once we've had a couple of coffees we can get going. However for some people this isn't an odd occurrence. This happens on a daily basis and sucks the energy from our very soul.

When we think of sleeping disorders we think of people who simply lie awake at night staring at the ceiling. This is more commonly known as insomnia this covers a whole spectrum variations. Some of these problems are easily treatable, some would have to be prevented by a doctor or specialized health professional. Some sleeping disorders can be extremely dangerous if they go undiagnosed for example sleep walking. Many people who suffer from these disorders face a lot of life threatening problems because having a sleeping disorder can disrupt you from living your normal everyday life.

This can fatigue someone to the point of exhaustion if they're spending more time worrying about their condition than getting the correct amount of sleep. The main problem with many people who are dealing with a sleeping disorder Is that they're not aware of it being a problem until they see it affecting their job and their everyday life. Those who suffer from this can also develop clinical depression because they feel like they're not able to do any of the things they're used to doing. They see it as a weakness and personal problem if they've been diagnosed with a sleep disorder.

**So what to do?**

Well we can go to a Doctor and he would give us a special test called the Polysomnogram which is used to determine and diagnose sleep disorders so specialists and doctors can plan a treatment designed for that individual person. Not all treatments are the same and will vary from person to person.

Common treatment options for sleeping disorders are:

- Behavioral/psychotherapeutic,
- Medications (Rozerem, Ambien, Ambien CR and Lunesta are common prescribed sleeping pills given for those diagnosed with a sleeping disorder), and
- Range of other somatic treatments that are given.
- People who have disorders such as narcolepsy usually have their brain activity measured to see where they are reaching peak points of sleeping so they can be treated since narcoleptics can't really work on jobs that require them to operate machinery or similar as they have to be alert and awake to know what they're doing.

The most common treatment to many people who are currently diagnosed with a sleeping disorder is usually treated medicinally for whatever time period the doctor prescribes and monitors the person's condition for. Having a sleeping disorder can make people feel like they're not normal. They can think they're sick but it's not a sickness and you can treat the problem through medicine and proper therapy to retrain your body to sleep on a normal scale.

**What is Average Sleep?**

Just how much sleep should we be having? The average person sleeps anywhere between 6-8 hours, but the most anyone sleeps is 10 hours. It's ideal to get the right amount of rest because of the fact that your immune system can lower when you don't get any kind of rest which can also trigger other medical and health issues from the lack of recovery. For me personally if I'm particularly busy with work and life in general have a number of late nights and early starts in a row I can suddenly feel lower on energy and I normally pick up a cold.

This can be a problem with mostly younger people because some lifestyles can acerbate the lack of sleep such as:

- Drug use
- Working long hours
- Drinking
- Smoking
- Poor diet consisting of a lot of unhealthy food choices
- Lack of exercise and maintaining physical health

## 2.  How to Tell If You Have a Sleep Disorder

Many people that have an undiagnosed sleep disorder. Friends or relatives may tell them they look very tired. They may experience mood changes, irritability or become overly emotional. Often they have difficulty paying attention, concentrating, or remembering things that are important. These are all symptoms of sleep deprivation, and possibly of a sleep disorder.

If you asked a person with an undiagnosed sleep disorder "What is the problem with your sleep?" You would usually receive the following answers.

1. "I have trouble falling asleep."
2. "I have trouble staying awake."
3. "I can't get up in the morning."
4. "I seem to do strange things in my sleep"
5. "I can't sleep because of my partner."

The specific answer chosen helps to narrow down the possibility of a precise type of sleep disorder.

When someone says "I can't fall asleep" it can mean several things. There could be a key issue when first going to bed, after waking up in the middle of the night, or in the early morning hours.

Many people suffer from not being able to fall asleep when they go to bed. This is called Sleep Latency. Sleep Latency can be a very serious symptom of certain sleep disorders, including sleep onset insomnia, delayed sleep phase disorder, shift work, restless leg syndrome or paradoxical insomnia.

Another problem people have is not being able to stay asleep, which is called Sleep Fragmentation. A person with this complaint can fall to sleep easily when they go to bed. However they wake up often throughout the night.

Other sleep disorders may include sleep maintenance insomnia, shift work. If a person wakes up very early in the morning and cannot get back to sleep, it could be a sign of advanced sleep phase disorder or sleep maintenance insomnia.

If the answer to the question is "I can't stay awake" and the person is falling asleep at inappropriate times they may be suffering from a sleep disorder such as Narcolepsy, obstructive or central sleep apnea, periodic limb movement disorder, restless leg syndrome, shift work or advanced sleep phase disorder.

People that say "I can't get up in the morning" and take an hour or more to fully wake from their sleep may suffer from excessive sleep inertia. They struggle making the transition from sleep to being awake. Sleep disorders that could be responsible for excessive sleep inertia are sleep apnea and delayed sleep phase disorder.

A person that answers the question with "I do strange things in my sleep" may find that their sleep is full of unexpected surprises. Sleepwalking, Sleep terrors, confusional arousals, REM sleep behavior disorder, nightmares, sleep-related eating disorder and bruxism are all types of sleep disorders known as parasomnias.

If a person answers "I can't sleep because of my partner" snoring, then this may actually be sleep apnea, bruxism, restless leg syndrome, or periodic limb movement disorder.

How would you answer the question of "What is the problem with your sleep?"

## 3. An Alternative Approach for Overcoming a Sleep Disorder

A sleep disorder can be very disruptive to everyday life and affects everything in our lives. Sleep deprived people are usually excessively tired and sleepy. They tend to become cantankerous and very emotional. Sometimes they become a danger, not only to themselves, but also to those around them.

There are a number of different natural strategies that people have found really beneficial. Some people use alternative, natural ways to lessen the effects of their sleep disorder. Many people focus on diet and nutrition, while others use herbs and supplements. Still others believe in the positive effect of exercise, relaxation and sensory techniques, meditation or behavioral and cognitive approaches. Often people use a combination of these approaches to help relieve the symptoms of their sleep disorder.

### Diet

A healthy diet is essential for optimal energy, and also provides a steady fuel source for us to do everything we want to do in our daily lives. Avoiding certain foods is as important as including others in your daily diet. The key is to eat a wide variety of foods and drink plenty of water to keep your body hydrated.

**If you're having trouble sleeping then look at your diet.**

How healthy is your diet? Do you drink a lot of sugary or energy drinks? Especially in the evening? A lot of cans of drink contain caffeine which is a stimulant and is great if it's a cup of coffee for perking you up in the morning. However energy drinks contain more than a cup of coffee and are loaded with sugar. This double whammy can really cause you problems if you drink these in the evening. This will certainly make getting sleep harder.

You want to avoid treated and processed foods that are high in salt – something which can dry you out and provide you with a restless night. Have you eaten a takeaway and woken up in the night needing a drink? That's the salt content drying you out.

In the reverse many foods promote restful sleep and are helpful in relieving some of the symptoms of certain sleep disorders. Eating the proper snack before bedtime can increase natural serotonin levels. Serotonin acts as a natural sedative and is made in the body from the amino acid tryptophan. Foods that are rich in tryptophan include chicken, turkey, cheese, cottage cheese, fish, milk, nuts, avocados and bananas.

Portion size is also important. If you work long hours you may push your main meal right to the point you get home which can be late. Then you're so hungry you have a large meal and then have trouble sleeping. The key is to have food prepared the day before and eat at the normal time. Don't eat more than you could fit on a cup saucer anywhere near bedtime. Something like yogurt would be a light choice.

**No Carbs**

Another great option to try out is no carbs at dinner time. This includes potatoes, rice, pasta, sweet potatoes, chips and bread. Your meal will probably becn some kind of meat and vegetable dish with salad. This is very light then. You could have a light snack later on if need be. Try this out, you'll be surprised how comfortable you feel.

**Herbs**

Many people have turned to herbs and natural supplements as an alternative approach to treating their sleep disorder. There are many nutritional supplements and herbal products on the market. It is key to know how a specific product acts on the body as well as on the specific sleep disorder. For example many people with restless leg syndrome have an iron or folic acid deficiency. Taking an iron supplement may alleviate some of the symptoms of RLS. Many herbs are well known for promoting a natural sleep. A clamming tea of chamomile or lemon balm can be very relaxing to many people that suffer from a sleep disorder.

## Exercise

I personally always get a much better night's sleep when I do some form of exercise during the day. A cardio workout before breakfast can really fire up the body for the day. It may seem impossible at first but I've gotten into a routine and I feel great. I then walk during the day and do some form of exercise later before dinner. A weights session after work before dinner can really get rid of the days tension. This really de-stresses the body and mind, it takes you away from your work and you just concentrate of the exercise at that moment.

## Meditation

Exercise and relaxation techniques, whether used alone or together, can reduce stress and muscle tension. Many people that use these techniques to lessen the symptoms of a sleep disorder do these before going to bed. They not only ease physical tension but they calm the mind and prepare the body to sleep. These techniques include mindful exercise, progressive muscle relaxation, breathing exercises and yoga. Perhaps a walk in the evening before or after dinner.

Meditation has become very popular as a form of alternative medicine. Visualization is also used by some sufferers of sleep disorders to calm the body before sleep. Two common forms of mediation are meditation on the breath and mantra meditation. Both of these types can have a positive effect on relieving stress and calming the body and mind. Many people focus their energy on a healing visualization as a method of alternative therapy for their sleep disorder and it can works really well.

**Sensory Techniques**

Hydrotherapy and aroma therapy are classed as sensory techniques. The two main techniques included in hydrotherapy, which means water therapy, are relaxing in an Epsom salt bath and a lymph stimulating footbath. Both are very relaxing. Aroma therapy includes the use of various therapeutic essential oils in baths, massage oils, room sprays, and simple inhalants.

**Alternative Strategies**

These are more about you changing things in your sleep routine, where you sleep, your bed clothes and even writing. Alternative behavioral and cognitive strategies used to combat the symptoms of a sleep disorder also include improving a person's sleep hygiene, stimulus control therapy and journal writing. Often they are used in conjunction with traditional medication and practices.

## 4. A Sleep Disorder That Affects the Legs - Restless Sleep Syndrome

Restless leg syndrome, known as RLS, is a sleep disorder that afflicts more than 15 percent of adults.

It affects more women than men and the incidence of restless leg syndrome tends to increase with age. Certain medical conditions, such as diabetes, arthritis and varicose veins, also increase the risk of developing restless leg syndrome.

This sleep disorder can vary from mild annoyance to being acutely painful. They are characterized by an uncontrollable urge to move the lower legs, knees and occasionally the arms. Sometimes painful sensations accompany the urge to move. People that suffer from this sleep disorder describe the feelings and sensations in different ways. Many describe a tingling, itching or pulling sensation. Still others say it feels prickly or burns. Some feel as if they have worms crawling under their skin.

The symptoms can cause the sufferer to get in and out of bed repeatedly which can delay or disrupt sleep. The sensations which are typical of this sleep disorder can occur anytime during the day or night. Restless leg syndrome occurring at night has a devastating effect on sleep.

The combination of always feeling tired and the symptoms themselves can cause a person with restless leg syndrome to alter their lifestyle. Long trips, movies, concerts and eating in restaurants are some of the activities they usually avoid. Attending a long meeting at work can become very painful and uncomfortable. People that have this sleep disorder can often suffer from depression.

Researchers believe that restless leg syndrome may be caused by malfunctions of the pathways in the brain that controls movement reflexes and sensations. Often this sleep disorder has a genetic base.

Restless leg syndrome cannot be diagnosed by one single test. Often standard neurological examinations show no signs of an abnormality. In many cases, a doctor makes the diagnosis of restless leg syndrome based on the description of the symptoms. They also take into account family history, and the results of a routine medical examination and blood tests.

Many times the treatment for restless leg syndrome is aimed at controlling the debilitating sensations that accompany this sleep disorder. Often iron supplements are prescribed because severe anemia has been linked to this disorder. Relaxation techniques, diet changes and the elimination of caffeine and alcohol help some sufferers of restless leg syndrome.

In most cases, this sleep disorder is treated with drugs. These drugs could include dopamine agents, benzodiazepines, opioids or anticonvulsants. Medications do not prevent restless leg syndrome, but they manage the symptoms. People that suffer from this sleep disorder usually have to stay on their medications for the rest of their lives.

Another sleep disorder similar to restless leg syndrome is periodic limb movement disorder known as PLMD. There are two main differences between restless leg syndrome and periodic limb movement disorder. Restless leg syndrome occurs when the sufferer is awake or asleep; intermittent limb movement disorder only occurs when the sufferer is asleep. Restless leg syndrome movements are voluntary responses to very unpleasant sensations; the movements of periodic limb movement disorder are involuntary and are not consciously controlled. Both of these sleep disorders can be successfully controlled with medical treatment.

## 5. Sleep Disorder - A Growing Concern in the United States

In the United States alone, it is estimated that approximately 60 - 80 million people have some form of sleep disorder. This number continues to rise year on year. Several of the reasons for the increasing numbers are the aging of the American population, the change in our lifestyle and the obesity epidemic. Of course there are other factors that can lead to a sleep disorder, such as, stress, shift work, illness or genetics.

As sleep disorders increase in the United States, so do the dangers that are associated with them.

Tiredness can lead to slower mental alertness and a slower reaction time. This can be a very dangerous combination. Between 20 - 25% of all serious vehicular accidents involve a tired driver. Many of these drivers suffer from some form of sleep disorder and may not even be aware of it. A large number of accidents that occur at home or at work are also due to people with some type of sleeping problem. Sleep disorder, combined with the cost of the accidents and associated illnesses it causes, results in the American people and the government spending billions of dollars.

Lack of sleep is directly related to many physical ailments and conditions. People that do not get sufficient sleep generally suffer headaches, sore joints and stomach problems. Often a sleep disorder is an underlying cause of heart problems, lung conditions and diabetes. Sleep disorders can also affect the mental well-being of people stricken with them. Mood changes, anxiety, eating disorders and depression can result.

Many people still do not think of a sleeping problem as a specific medical problem. Because of this, many never tell their physician that they are having a problem with sleep. Even if they see their doctor on a regular basis for an illness or condition, they never mention their difficulty sleeping. It seems trivial to the everyday person. But this is a mistake.

## Solutions

As the American public and medical community become more educated and aware of the symptoms, effects and severity of various sleep disorders, more and more cases are being diagnosed. Sufferers are being treated with medication, oxygen, cpap machines and even surgery in some cases.  There are better screening methods and diagnostic tests which find sleep disorder problems earlier. Overnight sleep centers no longer resemble a hospital room. They are now designed to look more like a hotel room, to make the patient feel more comfortable  In some cases, due to computerization and miniaturization, equipment can be so small that some testing can even be done at home.


Sleep is not an option or a luxury. It is a basic element of living and of good health. If you think you, your partner or your child may be suffering from a sleep disorder see your physician/Doctor. A sleep disorder is a medical problem that can be helped.

## 6. Sleep Disorder Affecting Shift Workers

This is a fairly common form of sleeping disorder among medical professionals, police officers, fireman and anyone else who works strange times. This is also attributed mostly to people who change their work schedules and sleeping times around frequently. You'll find this often in college students when they're changing semesters and quarters when they get new schedules and can sometimes throw sleep patterns off.

Meaning if you were used to getting up early one semester and then you get to sleep late on another it can throw your sleeping patterns off, which can make you feel unsettled and confused which is the main cause for why people get up and retire late, and are late for their jobs and classes because they're not giving themselves enough time to adjust between schedule changes.

This is why when a job or school schedules changes it's ideal to give yourself adequate time to make the adjustment so that it doesn't throw you off physically, so you're able to wake up and retire at a reasonable time so you can make it to work and school on time. The body likes to have a set pattern and we can plan appropriately.

This is why it's not always wise to constantly change your schedule whenever possible because if you do it too much you're going to confuse yourself on whether you're coming or going. There are some people whose jobs switch their schedules around so much that it can throw someone completely out of synch because the hours start to get rather conflicted when they're coming and going and not making time for other things like having a life or maintaining their priorities outside of their job and school. This can happen if you keep doing a late shift and your employer throws in an early shift once or twice a week. This can make sleep very hard.

This also can happen if you're running between more than one job and school because if you're going to a job during the day and then running to another job at night it can throw you off. People are advised to give themselves so much time between things in order to make the full transition into the new schedule or time frame so they're not feeling overwhelmed and stressed out since stress can play a huge thing in work related insomnia. The stress comes from having to make so many drastic changes too fast and at one time.

This is why people get burned out quickly and dealing with the physical things like indigestion and other things because they're pushing themselves too hard and sometimes forcing themselves to do things that isn't even normal and is considered unhealthy.

College students who are like this tending to gain or lose weight because of the stress they're under to switch from one thing to another and not giving themselves a chance to really adjust fully to a schedule or lifestyle change. Even people who work as nurses and doctors occasionally go through this. Because hours are rather strange, and that can throw off the pattern your body has become custom to when to rise and retire. If you interfere with that, it can make you feel peculiar which can also affect appetite and mental focus and concentration which most people deal with the disorientation of switching things around too fast. And as we've covered affecting appetite can also affect your mental and physical well-being and it becomes a vicious circle.

## 7. Sleep Disorder and Teenagers

There is a sleep disorder that affects between seven to ten percent of teenagers called Delayed Sleep Phase Disorder, also known as DNS.  Most teenagers outgrow this disorder by the time they reach young adulthood. Less then one percent of adults are believed to have DSP. People often mistake this sleep disorder for insomnia.

Left on their own, people with delayed sleep phase disorder would stay up until very late, sometimes right through to until 4 or 5 a.m. They like to get up very late in the morning or early afternoon. Often they are referred to as night owls.

Many teenagers like to stay up late and sleep late in the morning. Sometimes this is because they want to socialize at that time of the day. However, it can also be due to the likely delay in the circadian sleep / wake rhythm at their age of development.

Teenagers with this sleep disorder often have a very hard time getting up in the morning for school. Even if they go to sleep at a regular time, such as 11 p.m., they toss and turn for hours like someone with insomnia. They difference is, unlike an insomniac, people with delayed sleep phase disorder have no difficulty staying asleep. They do though have a very difficult time getting up early in the morning. Teenagers with this sleep disorder are very tired during the day and may even fall asleep in the classroom. The exact cause of this sleep disorder is not known. It is known for certain that it is a circadian rhythm problem.

Treatment for this sleep disorder is available for people that need to get onto a more traditional sleep / wake schedule. The types of treatment include, bright light, chronotherapy, melatonin and over-the-counter prescribed sleeping pills.

Bright light treatment for delayed sleep phase disorder uses a bright light to trick the brain's circadian clock. Exposure to bright light shifts the circadian rhythm if it is administered within a few hours of the body's lowest temperature at night.

Using chronotherapy as a treatment for someone with delayed sleep phase disorder requires a block of time one week long. Each day bedtime is delayed by three hours successively. For example, for someone that falls asleep at 2 a.m. but wants to fall asleep at 11. p.m., their bedtime would move to 5 a.m. on the first day. The next day it would move to 8 a.m. and continue this cycle for a week. A teenager suffering with delayed sleep phase disorder would need a week off from school in order to complete this therapy. Once the desired bed time is reached it is very important to keep a consistent wake up time.

There are numerous treatments involving various drugs that are used to treat delayed sleep phase disorder. Melatonin has been successful in changing the sleep cycle of people with this sleep disorder. Prescription medication such as Ramelteon, and other sleeping pills, have been successful in treating teenagers and adults with delayed sleep phase disorder.

If your teenager has trouble falling asleep and always wants to stay up late, be aware of the prospect that a sleep disorder may be present.

## 8. Nightmares - A Frightening Sleep Disorder

At some time in their childhood almost all children experience the sleep disorder of having a nightmare. They are more common in children and can begin as early as two years old. They are most common in children between three and twelve years old and are considered part of the normal developmental process. However, only about 3 percent, experience 'night terrors', also called sleep terrors. Both of these sleep disorders can be very frightening to a child.

Nightmares are dreams that are so frightening that they wake the person up. Everyone has had at least one nightmare in their life and they usually are not something to worry about. Nightmares occur several hours after going to sleep during the REM stage of sleep when there is general body paralysis and active dreaming.

Generally a child can remember the nightmare once they awake and they still remember it in the morning. Sometimes this nightmare sleep disorder can become a problem if the child has nightmares very often and becomes afraid to go to sleep or becomes sleep deprived. When a nightmare does occur it is important that the parent remains calm and reassuring.

There are several things that a parent can do to prevent nightmares. Discuss calm and comforting things with your child just before putting then to bed. Reading to them is a great way of relaxing them. A nice fairy tale, a positive upbeat adventure will take their mind away from the thought of the nightmare.

**Films and TV**

Don't let a child watch violent or scary shows on television, especially just before going to bed. These can have lasting effects when a child watches something that is too explicit for them to deal with on an emotional level. Maintaining a relaxing bedtime routine is also important. Sometimes, nightmares indicate a more severe emotional problem within your child.

**Night Terror**

Night terrors usually occur during the first few hours of sleep, during deep non-REM sleep. They often occur at the same time each night. Night terrors are characterized by screaming, crying or moaning. It is not unusual for a child experiencing a night terror to sit straight up in bed and scream. Their heart rate is rapidly increased and they experience intense breathing. An episode of this sleep disorder can last from 10 minutes to over an hour. Although the child's eyes are open, they are actually still asleep and when they wake up in the morning there is no memory of what happened during the night.

Although night terrors can be frightening, they are not dangerous. They usually are not a sign of any type of mental distress. A parent should not try to wake the child, or comfort them, during a night terror. The best thing for a parent to do when their child is experiencing a night terror is to make sure they are safe from falling out of the bed. Generally, most children outgrow this sleep disorder after a few months or years.

Several of the factors that can contribute to night terrors include being overly tired, staying up extremely late, eating a heavy meal just before going to bed, and taking certain medications.

Although nightmares and night terrors can seem like a very scary type of sleep disorder to both the parents and the children involved, they are generally harmless and the child should grow out of them.

## 9. Narcolepsy - The sleeping disease

Narcolepsy, a relatively rare sleep disorder, causes people to fall asleep when they do not want to. This is caused by a neurological disorder. The brain sends signals to the body that are sleep inducing; however, they are sent at inappropriate and unpredictable times. Often it happens when a person is involved in a quiet activity, such as watching a movie or during a meeting. Sometimes a person with this sleep disorder falls asleep while driving, which is obviously extremely dangerous. Others fall asleep while they are eating or talking. The overwhelming need to sleep can come at any hour of the day during any activity. Insomnia and fragmented sleep are a very common symptom of this sleep disorder. People with narcolepsey often have a very difficult time falling asleep at night, even though they fall asleep easily throughout the day. When they do fall asleep at night they wake up often and do not follow a typical REM / non REM sleep pattern.

Sleep paralysis occurs in about half of the people that suffer from this sleep disorder. For several minutes before falling to sleep or waking up, the person with this symptom cannot talk or move.

The loss of muscle function while awake is cataplexy. These episodes are usually very short in length.  Over half of the people with narcolepsy experience this symptom of this sleep disorder. They are caused by a part of REM not functioning correctly. Often, episodes are brought on by anger, laughter or any other strong emotion. Sometimes knees buckle, necks and jaws become weak or the person may fall to the ground. Even though the person looks like they are asleep and cannot talk, they are fully awake and aware of what is happening.

A hypnagogic hallucination is experiencing very vivid and often frightening sounds, images or physical sensations. These occur from dreams just before the person is falling asleep or waking up. It is very difficult for a person with this sleep disorder to distinguish between the dream and reality. These hallucinations often have very dangerous themes and are extremely frightening. Often they are accompanied by sleep paralysis.

There are also several lesser symptoms of narcolepsy. These include blurred vision, migraine headaches, memory or concentration problems and automatic behavior. An apostate of automatic behavior can last for several minutes. During that time a person with this sleep disorder will perform a routine task. The task is often done incorrectly, such as placing a turkey in the dishwasher or writing past the end of a page.

There are over 3 million cases of narcolepsy and is estimated by medical reports that 200,000 Americans are officially diagnosed by a doctor. It has been said that it's widespread like the neurological disease Parkinson's disorder. This condition is usually recognized in both men and women at any age, yet the symptoms are usually first noticed in teenagers and younger age adults usually in their 20s and early 30s.

It's been noted that there is a 15-year onset and actual diagnosis of the problem, which has contributed to the debilitating features of this particular disorder. Those who deal with narcolepsy have a plethora of cognitive, educational, occupational, and psychological issues that can arise from this problem. The presence of narcolepsy is 1 in 2000 people and is also found in people with diagnosed learning disabilities and currently the treatment options are very limited.

The studies that were conducted for this concluded that this problem is constantly under diagnosed in the general population in society. Some narcoleptics don't show any visible signs and the harshness of the condition varies from person to person.

**Tests**

Polysonogram and Multiple Sleep Latency exams are the two tests that are done to give a formal and correct diagnostic approach to the condition and usually this is where the diagnosis presents the level of severity so that it's properly noted by a specialist to ensure a proper treatment plan for that person. Tests are conducted in two-hour increments to allow the person to sleep and usually the polysonogram test does a continuous test of brain activity when it's in REM sleep mode when sleep happens at night.

People suffering with narcolepsy often do not realize how sleepy they are, nor how often they fall asleep. It is often a family member, friend or co-worker that convinces them that they need to seek medical help for their sleep disorder.

Narcolepsy has five main symptoms. These are excessive daytime sleepiness, insomnia and fragmented sleep, sleep paralysis, cataplexy and hypnagogic hallucinations. Some people with this sleep disorder experience only one symptom but others can experience all five.

Excessive daytime sleepiness is generally the first symptom to appear. Everyone with narcolepsy has this symptom. The feeling of needing to sleep is so strong that sufferers are unable to fend it off, regardless of how hard they try. These sleep attacks, as they are usually called, can happen several times and last for five to ten minutes.

Most narcoleptics fall asleep in night-time sleep mode fairly quickly. There are several methods of treatments for people with narcolepsy and usually it consists of anti-depressants and planned short-timed naps have also been helpful to lower the dependence on medicinal treatments and allowing the body to do what it should be doing naturally. Retraining the body to sleep at a reasonable time has helped those with narcolepsy to recognize sleeping at night and taking short naps during the day so that their body stays alert because a lot of narcoleptics have been putting themselves and others at risk when they fall asleep during their normal work day or even driving or operating machinery.

With the new wave of holistic medicine being readily available to help people with conditions from skin to psychological issues. Narcoleptics can also work with a treatment plan that includes a change in diet and incorporating exercise and taking nutritional supplements and formulas to give someone added nutrition if they're not getting enough from the food they eat.

Narcolepsy is very much manageable if you follow the doctor's instructions and taking medications when you're supposed to and following therapy plans that are designed for that person to follow to the last detail.

## 10.    Insomnia

Insomnia is the most common sleep disorder and affects about one third of the American population and is classified two different ways. It can be classified by how long it lasts - Transient insomnia lasts for only a few days, short term lasts for a few weeks and chronic lasts for more than three weeks.

The other way insomnia is classified is by its source. The main two classifications of this sleep disorder by source are primary and secondary.

### Transient insomnia

Transient insomnia is experienced by most people at some time throughout their lives. It can be caused by stress such as worrying about the first day school, an illness in the family, money troubles or needing to do something which will be very hard. Sometimes this sleep disorder occurs due to a disruption of their circadian cycle, which is a person's natural sleep cycle, caused by jet lag or a shift change at work. Transient insomnia goes away once the stress issue has passed. Short term insomnia is often caused by similar stressors as transient insomnia. If the sufferer of this sleep disorder cannot break the cycle of poor sleep, it often develops into chronic insomnia.

### Primary

Primary insomnia develops without any obvious cause. Sometimes it starts as early as infancy. Often it is the result of high metabolic rates or an overactive nervous system.

### Secondary

Secondary insomnia is the direct result of another cause. This sleep disorder can come from illness, medication, drugs or alcohol. Addressing the underlying cause of secondary insomnia often gives the sufferer relief. For example, if arthritis pain keeps you from sleeping, then treating the arthritis is the best way to cope with the poor sleep condition.

Insomnia is not a single disorder. It is a general symptom and could have many potential causes. In order to qualify as a sleep disorder, insomnia has to meet three specific requirements.

- First, the person has to experience poor sleep in general, or have a problem falling or staying asleep.
- Second, if given the proper sleep environment and an adequate opportunity to sleep, the problem still occurs.
- Third, the result of the poor sleep causes some type of impairment while awake. Examples of an impairment are; fatigue, body aches and pains, inability to concentrate, mood changes, lack of energy, poor concentration, or developing an unnatural amount of worry about sleep.

Often insomnia is treated with medication, such as sleeping pills. These can be prescription medication or bought over the counter.

However, there are several other methods of treatment for this sleep disorder:

Behavioral treatments include meditation, progressive muscle relaxation, deep breathing, visualization, biofeedback, sleep hygiene, cognitive behavioral therapy and reconditioning sleep restriction. These methods are often very successful.

Some sufferers of this sleep disorder choose holistic, or alternative, treatment. This method involves the use of herbal supplements which are not usually FDA approved. Others seek acupuncture as a way to relieve their insomnia.  Passive body heating, which is the use of hot baths is another method used.

Understanding this sleep disorder is the first step to breaking the cycle of insomnia.

**Inspiration**

Insomnia has been a featured disorder from many factors such as books and movies. It has inspired characters who are usually jaded with society or have other issue and the insomnia is used to draw attention to that. This seems to be the most common form of sleeping disorder to the point that movies and songs were made about this problem.

People aren't aware that this is a problematic issue for those who suffer from this. It's not healthy to go without sleep because it can affect your immune system making you prone to catching things like the flu and colds. Not getting any rest can cause severe disorientation because your body wasn't given an opportunity to rest and recuperate.

This is what drove the designer coffee movement up like the sprawl of coffee shops from Starbucks, Costa etc since you had a lot of late nighters consisting of mainly people working in hospitals and college students who had to pull late nighters and cram sessions needed to stay awake.  When coffee wasn't working they bought this over the counter pill called Vivarin which is equal to about 2 cups of coffee when you take the prescribed dosage.

It's usually not a good idea to take Vivarin because it can interfere with your body's ability to sleep and rest normally. You'll find more college students getting sick a lot because they're forcing their bodies to do things that isn't normal like staying up super late and not getting at least 6 hours of sleep.

## It's good to rest

Rest allows your body's digestive system respite which makes up about 70% of your immune system so it's ideal to sleep when necessary and taking short naps also work as a re-energizer to give you a burst of energy that works much better than coffee or caffeine pills.

You can actually build up a resistance to caffeine. A lot of coffee drinkers tend to get very tired after a certain point and that's due in part to the fact that you build up a resistance after having a few cups of coffee or cans of Coke so meaning it won't keep you awake as long. In fact it will accelerate the rate of how fast you'll start to feel sleepy.

Seeing pop culture idolize such a disorder is unknown unless the person who wrote the book or penned the song has a problem with it and decided to write or sing about it. The reason for it is unknown, but it's rather fascinating since a song can tell a story and the same of a book, but it's obviously influenced a slew of songs, movies books and computer games where the characters are suffering from some kind of sleeping disorder from mild to severe.

## 11.     Hypersomnia - Oversleeping

Most people don't realize they oversleep when they have a condition called hypersomnia and that's due in part to recurring episodes of excessive daytime sleeping and prolonged night-time sleep. This is different from the average person taking that midday nap. Hypersomnia can be done at the most inappropriate times like at work, during meals, or even in conversation with people.

Hypersomniacs are also diagnosed with narcolepsy, which can be quite dangerous because some individuals are behind the wheel of cars or even cooking in their home and aren't aware that they fell asleep. Some hypersomniacs and narcoleptics can fall asleep and then wake up and resume where they left off in conversations with people. Usually daytime naps usually provide no relief or symptoms to the problem and will result in the individual having increased difficulty in waking from a long extended period of sleeping: disorientation, anxiety, decreased energy, increased fatigue, restlessness, slow thinking, slow speech, loss of appetite, hallucinations, and problems with memory functions.

Some individuals also experience losing the ability to function in normal family, social, occupational, and other settings familiar to that person.

Hypersomnia can be triggered by sleep apnea or narcolepsy, where it can lead to dysfunction of the autonomic nerve system, which can be brought on, by acute alcohol and/or drug abuse. In some cases rare or not it can also be triggered from physical problems such as tumors, head trauma or injuries to the nervous system. Specific medications or withdrawal of medications and/or drugs may contribute to someone having hypersomnia. Medical conditions such as multiple sclerosis, depression, encephalitis, epilepsy, and obesity can contribute to hypersomnia as well.

It's also been noted that those who have hypersomnia are also genetically dispositioned to this problem whereas in others there's no known or documented cause. Hypersomnia typically affects adolescents and young adults in their 20s and 30s. Although the most common causes of this disorder differs in the age brackets. Information can be located on the National Institute of Neurological Disorders and Strokes website if you're looking for a more thorough clinical explanation to this problem. This isn't a substitute for medical advice from a licensed physician so it's ideal to educate yourself first. But leave the diagnosing and treatment to a doctor so that you condition can be monitored closely.

People who are not seeing a doctor when they identify problems that are not normal for them to experience are misdiagnosing too many issues with sleep. Persons who are severely obese can also have a difficult time losing the weight because of the fact that lack of sleep can increase the body's metabolic rate, which can trigger excessive hunger In those who are trying to lose weight.

This is why so many people who are obese are eating more than they should because a lot of them sleep so much that they wake up wanting to eat when they should be sleeping like normal people do and not up at all hours of the night wanting to eat. This is why it's harder for people who are obese to lose weight when they sleep too much and not training their body to rest instead of wanting to eat food. This can be a vicious circle but once you've found the problem, you can follow the steps your Doctor prescribes.

## 12.    Fatal Familial Insomnia

This is one of the rarest forms of sleeping disorders that we know of. This is an inherited disorder that has only been found in 28 families in the world that have the dominant gene for it. The offspring of a parent of developing the disorder is about 50% and there is no cure for this. The age of onset is around the ages between 30 and 60 and the disorder's time frame runs between 7 to 18 months.

This disease has 4 stages that it goes through and 1st stage of the disease starts off with the sufferer dealing with increased insomnia leading to severe panic attacks, and various kinds of phobias. This stage lasts about 4 months.

The 2nd stage sufferer deals with hallucinations and panic attacks become more obvious and lasts about 5 months.

3rd stage leads to total inability to sleep. And follows with drastic weight loss and lasts about 3 months.

4th stage Dementia sets in and progressively becoming irresponsive and mute over a course of 6 months and this is the final progression of the disease.

This sounds a lot like Alzheimer's because if you notice the time frame it's a lot less shorter than the actual time span of someone who deals with Alzheimer's because the sufferer is dealing with it for several years instead of a year where the disease progressively degenerates the mental capacity to such a degree that the sufferer has a hard time with memory.

As far as treatment is concerned sleeping pills don't have any effect for people suffering from Fatal Familial Insomnia and not even non-medicinal therapy can work either. Medical science has no idea why it's a fatal disease and how they can create effective treatment options to combat this problem. And more effective genetic testing for diseases that are inherited to find out what can be done medicinally and therapeutically to deal with this sleeping disorder.

It's a matter of how much attention the medical world takes note of this and pushes the funding to finding a cure and effective genetic testing of families and tracking diseases through the generations to be able to have some kind of record of the disease passing down through generations or skipping generations which is what some ailments have done in some families for those who have a disposition for certain things.

This doesn't get nearly as much attention as all the other sleeping disorders because of it being rare, and only turning up in so many people and births making it not rare enough for it to get the recognition as regular insomnia and to qualify for the treatments. That are currently out there to help those 60 million people who are dealing with some kind of sleeping disorder.

With the way medical science is going it will be a matter of time before medical science catches up and helps the many people who are looking for a cure of being deprived of a restful night's sleep. The moment a cure is found is one less person having a poor night's sleep and it's a step closer to living a normal life.

## 13.      Children and Sleepwalking

The sleep disorder of sleepwalking, also known as
somnambulism, affects approximately 14% of school-age
children between five and twelve years old at least once in their
life. Approximately one quarter of the children with this sleep
disorder have more frequent episodes. Sleepwalking is more
common in boys then it is in girls. Most children that sleepwalk
mature from the symptoms of this sleep disorder by
adolescence as their nervous systems develop.

In children this sleep disorder is thought to be the result of the
immaturity of the brain's sleep / wake cycle. Normally the
entire brain wakes up at the same time. However, in the case
of a sleepwalker, the entire brain does not wake up together.
The portion that is responsible for mobility wakes up while the
portion responsible for cognition and awareness stays asleep.
So this actually means the child sis in a deep state of sleep.

With this sleep disorder the brain remains partially asleep but
the body is able to move. It is common for the sleepwalker to
get out of bed and walk around. Sometimes they get dressed or
go outside. Even though the sleepwalker's eyes are open and
they see what they are doing, their expression remains
blank.They do not respond to conversation or even to their
name being called. A sleepwalker's movements usually appear
clumsy. It is not uncommon for them to trip over furniture or
knock over things as they move around. A sleepwalking episode
usually happens one to two hours after the child goes to sleep.
Most of these episodes last for fifteen minutes or less, but some
can last for an hour or more.

This sleep disorder in children is usually outgrown and
treatment is not generally necessary. In most cases, a parent

gently guiding the child back to bed is all that is needed. There is not any need to wake the child as you'll startle them.

However, there is about 1% of the population that sleepwalk as adults. Adults that have this sleep disorder did not necessarily have it as a child. In adults a sleepwalking episode can be triggered by stress, anxiety, sleep fragmentation, sleep deprivation, or certain medical conditions such as epilepsy.

Treatment for adults with this sleep disorder is often reliant on upon the amount of danger they are in during an episode. For example, a sleepwalker who opens doors and goes outside onto a busy city street is in danger. A sleepwalker that gets up and goes into the living room and sits down on a chair most likely is not in danger. Treatments can include behavioral therapies, self-hypnosis, or prescription medication.

A sleepwalker, whether adult or child, needs to have a safe area so that they do not get hurt during an episode. Precautions can be taken to eliminate some dangers. Parents should make sure the child's bedroom does not have any sharp or breakable objects. Doors should be locked at night to keep the sleepwalker from going outside. Sometimes it is necessary to put bells on doors to alert the sleeping parent that their child is actually sleepwalking. Large glass windows and doors should be covered with heavy drapery to lessen the chance of having the sleepwalker walk through it while it is closed.

## Somnambulism

A child with the sleep disorder of somnambulism needs to be protected and kept safe during an episode. It is the environment they are in that is the danger more than the sleep disorder itself.

## 14.    Medications Used for the Sleep Disorder of Chronic Insomnia

People that suffer from the sleep disorder of chronic insomnia must decide whether or not they are going to take a sleep medication. This decision is usually made with their Doctor/physician. Many people decide to take a sleeping pill because it offers relief from the symptoms of their sleep disorder and the extreme sleepiness they are always feeling. Taking a pill can improve how they feel and also the quality of their life. However, many people worry about the side effects and health risks that come with taking sleeping pills. Sleeping pills are among the most widely used drugs in the United States, and their use continues to escalate.

The types of sleep medications that are available to people with insomnia fall into two categories, prescription and over-the-counter medications. Each sleep medication affects the body differently. The effectiveness of the sleeping pill is a major factor when dealing with sufferers of this sleep disorder. How quickly the pill will take effect and how long the effect will last are very important. The effect should equal the individual's sleep problem. The fast acting drugs would benefit a person who has difficulty falling asleep while a longer lasting pill would better benefit someone who has difficulty staying asleep.

Other important factors concerning medications for people with this sleep disorder include the impact the medication has on sleep quality, the tolerance that a person has for the drug, the possibility of developing a dependence on the drug, and the side effects associated with said drug. Each of these points has to be considered when deciding to take sleep medication for chronic insomnia.

Many over-the-counter sleep medications contain some type of antihistamine as a primary active ingredient. Antihistamines are widely used to treat allergies and they are also effective in helping people fall asleep. However, there has been little research done on their long-term effectiveness or safety.

Prescription medications for the sleep disorder of chronic insomnia are classified into four general groups: benzodiazepine receptor agonists, antidepressants, melatonin receptor agonists, and barbiturates. Each one of these drug groups has specific benefits in regards to treating insomnia. However, it is very important that the right type of for chronic insomnia medication is prescribed for each individual person with this sleep disorder.

Before choosing a sleeping medication, it is very important to determine the source of the insomnia. For example, perhaps the source of the insomnia is the result of another treatable illness, or a side effect of a medication that is taken. The insomnia is then called secondary insomnia. The focus on medication should then be on the primary illness. Cure the primary problem and you should in turn cure the sleeplessness. Often the insomnia will disappear once the underlying cause is treated.

The decision of whether or not to take sleep mediation for chronic insomnia has to be a personal decision. There is no right or wrong decision. However, it is important, if the choice is to take a medication for this sleep disorder, to become as educated as possible about the medication prescribed.

## 15.     Muscle pain and sleeplessness

Fibromyalgia is a painful condition that affects the muscles and joints and is seen in only 3-6% of the general population in the world. It's generally seen more in females than males with a ratio percentage of 9.1 according to the College of Rhumatology and is commonly diagnosed in females between the ages of 20-50. It's been noted that the onset happens in childhood. This is not a life-threatening disease though the degree of pain in the condition can vary day to day with periods of flare ups and remission. The disease is being argued and viewed as non-progressive, but that's a point that remains in an indeterminate state.

This is a problematic issue that can be a reason to keep someone up at night because the pain can be unbearable with the tingling and achiness in the muscles. This drives many who deal with this to endless and chronic deprivation of sleep. Those who suffer fibromyalgia also note issues with memory and other neurological issues, but the most frequent is the issues with sleeping that individuals go through when they deal with painful, annoying outbreaks.

Other issues that surround this problem, which can make sleeping very difficult, are irritable bowel syndrome with constipation, which affects mostly women and few men. Skin disorders like dermatological disorders, headaches, myofacial twitching, and symptomatic hypoglycemia. Stress, excessive physical exertion, lack of sleep, changes in temperature and baromic pressure. This condition can worsen when individuals don't sleep or getting the proper rest and not overdoing on things in their daily lives.

The American Medical Association had officially recognized fibromyalgia as a medical condition back in 1987 when the disorder was around since the 1800s. It's been said that flare ups are not identical to the ones that are found in people with rheumatoid arthritis.

Ibuprofen like Advil, Acenomenofen (Tylenol), and Neproxine (Aleve) which are anti-inflammatory and can bring some comfort to those with fibromyalgia flare ups. Massage has also been useful in helping those who deal with fibromyalgia to find comfort when they have flare ups. Massage helps to transfer fluids from the muscles and joints and increases circulation to the affected areas to bring some temporary relief for soreness and flare ups.

It's best to get a massage when you're not on any medication due to the high risk of side effects that can be triggered from massaging tissue and muscles.

Fibromyalgia is a manageable problem if you follow your doctor's instructions and take your medication as directed and getting the right amount of sleep and getting plenty of exercise. Eating a nutritious diet consisting of fresh fruits and vegetables and drinking plenty of water can also make vast improvements to the condition.

Likewise limiting things in the diet that can also aggravate flare ups. Your Doctor can help with the foods than can cause problems for you. When you take care of yourself properly you can actually improve the quality of sleep as well as decreasing the debilitating pain.

All these things can help assist you with a good night's sleep and avoid keeping you up all night long. Once you get a good night's sleep, you will rest and feel more stress free and more relaxed, so that you can face the day with no painful flare ups and discomfort that can be annoying.

## 16.        Sleep Disorder Overnight Sleep Center

A new option if you think you may have a sleep disorder that your primary doctor or a doctor that specializes in sleep disorders can now send you to a sleep center for diagnosis. There are a large number of sleep centers located across the United States and the world and their numbers are increasing. Sleep centers in the United States must be accredited by the American Academy of Sleep Medicine.

When a person goes to a sleep center, it is usually for an overnight stay.  Costs involved for most sleep study tests range from one to three thousand dollars and many need to be repeated twice. The first visit to establish the sleep disorder and the second to get accurate settings for any PAP machines that may be needed. Health insurance generally pays all or most of the cost of the tests needed to diagnose a sleep disorder.

Once an appointment has been made, many sleep centers send a sleep diary to the patient.  The information from the sleep diary is used by the doctors to understand general sleeping patterns.

As you can imagine it is also recommended that no caffeine or alcohol be consumed after 12:00 p.m. on the day of the scheduled test. Generally the patient packs an overnight bag just as if they were going to stay at a hotel overnight. During the sleep study you wear your own nightclothes and you can use a favorite pillow from home. You can bring a book or magazine if you like to read before falling to sleep.

Most sleep centers resemble a hotel room and have a television to watch if that is what the patient usually does before going to sleep at home. Once you are relaxed the sleep center technician starts preparation for the equipment needed to record your patterns of sleep.

Diagnosis from a sleep center study is made using polysomnography which records a continual record of your sleep. In order to take a specific reading slightly more than two dozen small thin electrodes are pasted to specific parts of your body.

They are placed:

- under your chin,
- on your scalp,
- near your eyes and nose,
- on your finger,
- chest and legs,
- and also over the rib muscles and on the abdomen.

These electrodes then record various types of readings during the night. Often an audio and video tape are also made to monitor sleep noises and movement.

Once all the equipment is in place the sleep technician leaves you alone to fall asleep. Even with all the equipment it is not uncomfortable. It is easy to move or turn onto your side. Each bedroom in a sleep center also has an automatic intercom so it is easy to call the technician if needed for such things as a bathroom break. When the sleep study is completed, the specialist may wake you. Most studies that are used to diagnose a sleep disorder take seven to eight hours.

The information is collected on a computer file called a polysonagram and are monitored and analyzed by the sleep technician during the night. The results are then sent for further readings to determine if there is a sleep disorder.

Although a sleep study may not sound comfortable, it is very important to determine and treat any sleep disorder.

## 17.     12 Cures To Get Great Sleep

Here is a quick check list to aid your sleep:

### 1. Set a sleep schedule—and stick with it

If you do only one thing to improve your sleep, this is it, says Dr. Daniels: Go to bed at the same time every night and get up at the same time every morning—even on weekends. A regular sleep routine keeps your biological clock steady so you rest better.

### 2. Keep a sleep diary

To help you understand how your habits affect your rest, track your sleep every day for at least 2 weeks. Write down not only what's obviously sleep related—

- what time you go to bed,
- how long it takes you to fall asleep,
- how many times you wake up during the night,
- how you feel in the morning

Also factors like what you ate close to bedtime and what exercise you got.

### 3. Stop smoking

Nicotine is a stimulant, so it prevents you from falling asleep. Plus, many smokers experience withdrawal pangs at night. Smokers are 4 times more likely not to feel as well rested after a night's sleep than non-smokers. Smoking exacerbates sleep apnea and other breathing discord.

### 4. Review your medications

What are you already taking? Beta-blockers (prescribed for high blood pressure) may cause insomnia; so can SSRIs (a class of antidepressants that includes Prozac and Zoloft).

### 5. Exercise, but not within 4 hours of bedtime

Working out is great for you, especially cardio improves the length and quality of your sleep, says Dr. Daniels. That said, 30 minutes of vigorous aerobic exercise keeps your body temperature elevated for about 4 hours and can really affect sleep.

### 6. Cut caffeine after 2 pm

That means coffee, tea, cola and all energy drinks. Caffeine is a stimulant that stays in your system for about 8 hours.

### 7. Write down your woes

Every night jot down your top concerns, things that you are thinking about, things you need to do tomorrow, Then write down the steps you can take to solve the problems, a 'to-do' list. This positive plan of attack will help you to stop worrying, you know what you need to do tomorrow.

### 8. Take time to wind down

You need to give your body time to unwind. You can't just jump into bed having been closely texting on your tablet for the past hour.  Give your body time to transition from your active day:

### First 20 minutes:

Prep for tomorrow (pack your bag, set out your clothes).

### Next 20:

Take care of personal hygiene (brush your teeth, moisturize your face).

### Last 20:

Relax in bed, practicing deep breathing, light reading with a low light, but don't use your mobile or tablet, it will activate your brain to get working again.

### 9. Sip milk, not a martini

It takes an average person about an hour to metabolize one drink, so if you have two glasses of wine with dinner, finish your last sip at least 2 hours before bed.

### 10. Snack on cheese and crackers

The ideal night-time nibble combines carbohydrates and either calcium or a protein that contains the amino acid tryptophan, studies show that both of these combos boost serotonin, a naturally occurring brain chemical that helps you feel calm.

### 16. Eliminate light sources

The glow from your laptop, iPad, smart phone, or any other electronics on your nightstand may pass through your closed eyelids and retinas into your hypothalamus—the part of your brain that controls sleep.

### 14. Spray a sleep-inducing scent

Certain smells, such as lavender, chamomile, and ylang-ylang, activate the alpha wave activity in the back of your brain, which leads to relaxation and helps you sleep more soundly. Mix a few drops of essential oil and water in a spray bottle and give your pillowcase a light spray.

### 18. Check your pillow position

The perfect prop for your head will keep your spine and neck in a straight line to avoid tension or cramps that can prevent you from falling asleep. Ask your spouse to check the alignment of your head and neck when you're in your starting sleep position.

### 20. Stay put if you wake up

If you don't feel anxious or uncomfortable then stay put, just relax and breathe deeply.

## Conclusion

We have reached the end of my book on 'Sleep' and I truly hope you have found this useful. Getting a good night's sleep can be life-changing when all you've experienced is poor sleep. There are a lot of things you can do immediately from your diet to cutting out energy drinks to doing more exercise. These are very simple remedies.

Please leave a review on amazon as they help me carry on and write more books like this.


All the best

M

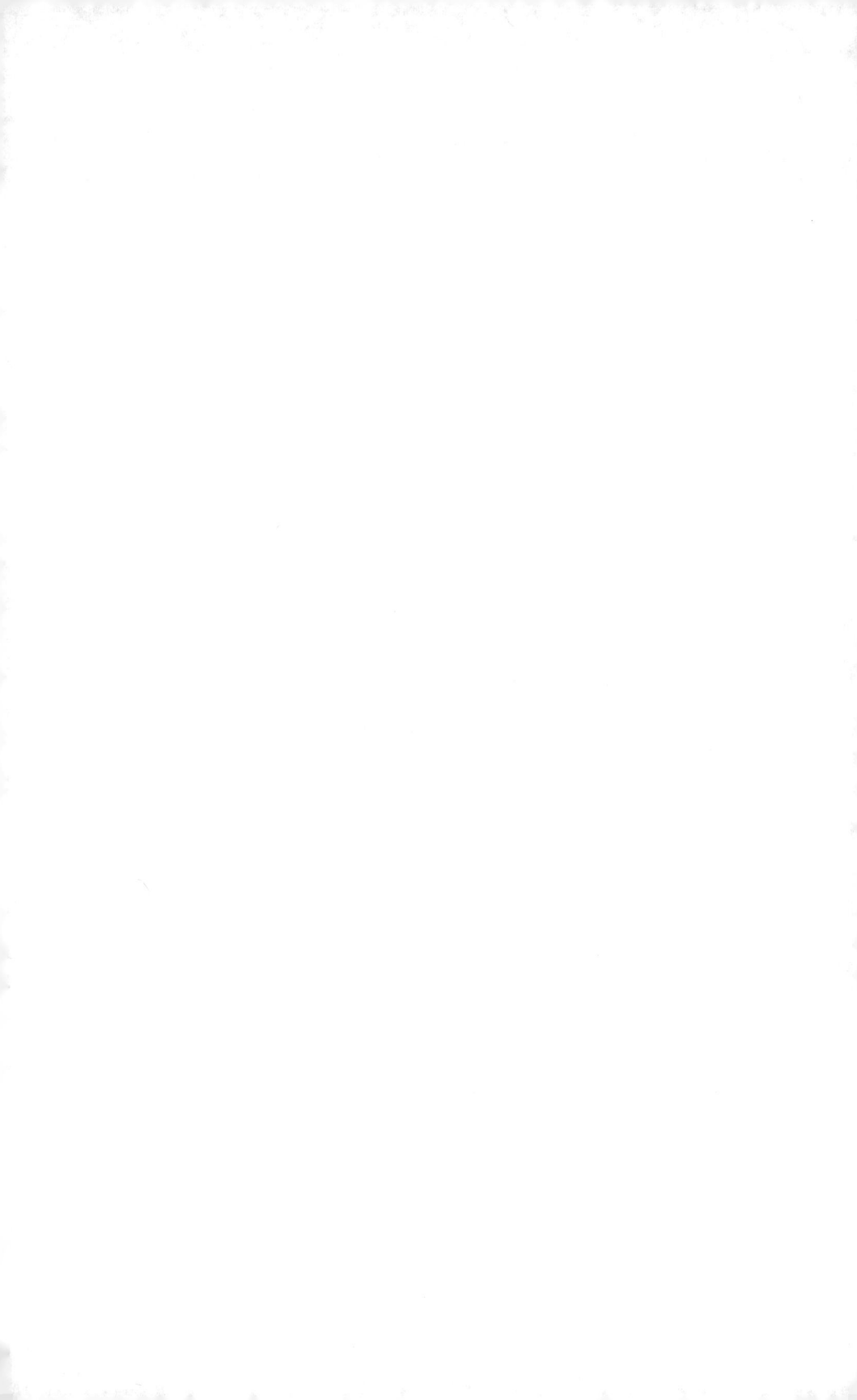

www.ingramcontent.com/pod-product-compliance
Lightning Source LLC
Chambersburg PA
CBHW060650290526
45793CB00001B/473